Publish

Bulletproof Diet Cookbook: Quick and Easy Bulletproof

Diet Recipes to Lose Weight and Increase Energy by

Following the Bulletproof Diet

ISBN 978-1-990120-84-8

TABLE OF CONTENTS

Original Bulletproof Coffee

Ingredients:

- 2 Tbsp. Of Butter, unsalted and Grass Fed
- 2 Tbsp. Coconut Oil
- 2 Cups of Coffee, Hot Brewed and Made With Low Toxin Beans

Directions:

1. Brew your coffee mixture as you normally would, but make sure that you use a metal filter if you can.
2. While you coffee is brewing add some hot water into a blender. After your coffee brews pour out the hot water and add your freshly brewed coffee, butter and coconut oil into your blender.

3. Cover your blender and blend your coffee until there is a little layer of foam on the top of your mixture.
4. Pour into serving cups and add a dash of cinnamon, dark chocolate, sweetener or vanilla if you want.

Minty Avocado Smoothie

Ingredients:

- 1 cup coconut milk
- 1 tablespoon erythritol
- 1 tablespoon colostrum powder
- 1 small avocado, peeled and pitted
- 4 mint leaves

Directions:

1. Combine all the Ingredients: in a blender and pulse until smooth and creamy.
2. Serve the smoothie as fresh as possible.

Chicken With Pesto, Vegetables And Fresh Cheese

Ingredients:

- 1 tomato
- A sachet of sautéed vegetables
- A bowl of cream cheese
- 300 g chicken
- 1 tablespoon pesto

Directions:

1. Cook the chicken and cover with pesto on both sides.
2. Cook the vegetables.
3. Cut the chicken into pieces, add the vegetables and tomatoes and mix.
4. Add fresh cheese to your taste.

Grass Fed Sirloin Steak, Macadamia Dressing, Raw Asparagus Salad

Ingredients:

- 1 teaspoon fresh thyme leaves
- Juice of 1 lemon
- ½ garlic clove, minced
- Salt and pepper to taste
- 2 grass fed sirloin steaks
- 3 cups asparagus
- 6 tablespoons coconut oil
- ½ cup macadamia nuts

Directions:

1. Lightly heat griddle.
2. Shave asparagus with a speed peeler into ribbons and set aside in a bowl.

3. Take a small blender and add the macadamia nuts, half the coconut oil, thyme leaves and lemon juice.
4. Roughly blend and season with salt. Set aside.
5. Rub the rest of the coconut oil over the steak and season with salt and pepper.
6. Add to the griddle and cook to your liking. For a thick steak cook around 4 minutes each side for medium rare.
7. Once steak is cooked, take out and leave to rest. While steak is resting pour the macadamia dressing on a plate and add the raw asparagus ribbons on top.
8. Slice the steak and serve on top of the dressing and salad.

Basic Butter Bulletproof Coffee

Ingredients:

- 1 tbsp MCT oil
- 2 tbsp unsalted butter
- 1 cup newly prepared coffee

Directions:

1. Combine every one of the fixings in a blender and continue to process until smooth.
2. Pour into a glass and enjoy!

Highoctane Coffee Or Tea

Ingredients:

- 12 T grassfed butter
- 12 T coconut oil
- 2 cups lowtoxin brewed coffee (or green tea)

Directions:

1. While the coffee is brewing, put hot water in a glass blender to preheat it.
2. When you're ready to make your highoctane coffee, empty the water.
3. Put all the Ingredients: into the blender.
4. Put the lid on with a kitchen towel over it.
5. Holding the lid down with your hand (and the towel), blend the beverage until you have a nice froth on the top. [You can use an immersion or hand blender but it won't mix as well.]

6. Pour into your mug and drink somewhat slowly to give your body time to process the oils.

Avocado And Mushroom Breakfast

Ingredients:

- 2 tablespoons grass fed butter or ghee
- Salt to taste
- Pepper powder to taste
- Fresh herbs of your choice to garnish
- 1 medium avocado, peeled, pitted, sliced
- 2 large pastured eggs
- 4 large Portobello mushrooms
- 6 high quality pastured bacon slices

Directions:

1. Place a nonstick skillet over medium low heat. Add half the butter.

2. Place the mushrooms with its topside down. Sauté until mushrooms are tender. Sprinkle salt and pepper over it.
3. Remove from heat and transfer on to a serving platter.
4. Place the pan back on heat and add the remaining butter. Add bacon. Crack the eggs in it and cook until done.
5. Remove on to the serving platter.
6. Serve with avocado slices.

Frozen Almond Bulletproof Coffee Smoothie

Ingredients:

- 1 cup of almond milk, or of choice
- ½ tsp. of raw organic milk
- 2 tbsp. of Bulletproof coffee, of choice
- 2 frozen organic bananas, chopped
- ½ cup of raw honey, or less

Directions:

1. Prepeel and chop the organic bananas and place them in a freezer bag four hours prior.
2. Once the chopped organic bananas are frozen, place them into a blender along with the other Ingredients:.
3. Blend the mixture until it is smooth and even.

Simple Bone Broth

Ingredients:

- ½ cup of oregano, rosemary, thyme and sage, fresh and roughly chopped
- 1 to 2 tablespoons of vinegar, apple cider variety
- 1 cup of broth, optional and beef variety
- Dash of sea salt, for taste
- 3 carrots, fresh, medium in size and cut into small sized pieces
- 3 stalks of celery, cut into small sized pieces
- 2 ½ pounds of beef marrow bones, grass fed variety

Directions:

1. Using a large sized stockpot, add in your carrots and celery. Set over medium heat and cook for the next 5 to 10 minutes or until translucent.
2. Then add in your beef marrow bones, your rosemary, thyme, oregano and fresh sage. Cover with some warm water and stir to combine.
3. Add in your vinegar and allow to simmer over low heat for the next 8 to 14 hours.
4. Once your broth is deep brown in color, remove your bones from your broth and strain your veggies out.
5. Season with some more salt and serve whenever you are ready.

Poached Eggs With Some Sautéed Greens

Ingredients:

- 2 eggs, poached
- 2 tbsp. Of almonds, sliced finely
- 2 to 3 cups of kale and collards, freshly and washed
- 2 tbsp. Of butter, unsalted and grass fed
- Dash of sea salt for taste

Directions:

1. Fill a medium sized pan with about an inch or so of water. Add in your mixed greens to cook over medium heat. Cook your greens until they become tender. Drain your water.
2. Next add in your butter and toss your greens gently until completely covered. Remove your greens from heat.

3. Sprinkle your greens with some salt and nuts and toss again to cover. Top with your poached eggs and serve immediately.

Lemon Green Tea Smoothie

Ingredients:

- 1/2 cup coconut milk
- 1 tablespoon erythritol
- 1 tablespoon MCT oil
- 2 tablespoons lemon juice
- 1 tablespoon organic Matcha powder
- 1 cup coconut water

Directions:

1. Mix all the Ingredients: in a blender and pulse until smooth.
2. Pour the drink in glasses and serve it as fresh as possible.

Salmon And Spinach Eggs

Ingredients:

- 4 eggs
- 1 teaspoon of herbs of your choice
- ½ red pepper
- 450 g frozen spinach with cream
- 400 g pink salmon

Directions:

1. Preheat the oven to 175 degrees.
2. Mix all the Ingredients:.
3. Pour into muffin tins, almost to the edge.
4. Bake for about 15 minutes.

Steamed Fillet Of Haddock With Fennel, Lemon & Parsley

Ingredients:

- Juice of 2 lemons
- 3 tablespoon coconut oil
- Salt and pepper to taste
- 2 fillets of haddock
- 2 cups fennel, finely sliced
- ¼ cup flat leaf parsley, chopped

Directions:

1. Place fillets of haddock in bamboo steamer and cook for around 810 minutes.
2. Add the fennel, lemon juice, parsley and salt and pepper to a bowl with the coconut oil. Mix well.

3. Serve the salad on a plate on top of the haddock fillets.

Vanilla Cream Bulletproof

Ingredients:

- 1 tsp vanilla extract
- 1 tbsp without sugar maple syrup
- 1 tbsp unsalted butter
- 1 ¼ cups newly fermented coffee
- 1 tbsp MCT oil
- 2 tbsp weighty cream

Directions:

1. Process every one of the fixings in a blender until smooth.
2. Fill a spotless glass and enjoy.

Avodeviled Eggs

Ingredients:

- 1 T organic shallot, minced
- ½ tsp. celery seed (optional)
- Sea salt (to taste)
- Organic paprika (to garnish)
- 8 hardboiled eggs
- 1/2 large ripe avocado, mashed
- 1 tsp. raw apple cider vinegar

Directions:

1. Slice the eggs in half lengthwise and gently pop the yolks into a bowl.
2. Add the avocado, vinegar, shallot, and celery seed.
3. Mash and mix until well combined.

4. Add salt to taste. Spoon or pipe the mixture into the egg halves and garnish with a sprinkle of paprika.

Gluten Free Pancakes

Ingredients:

- ½ tablespoon ground flaxseed
- ¼ teaspoon baking soda
- ¼ teaspoon sea salt
- 1 tablespoon coconut oil or grass fed unsalted butter melted + extra for greasing
- 1 ½ cups almond meal
- 6 tablespoons almond milk, unsweetened
- 2 small pastured eggs

Directions:

1. Whisk together eggs and almond milk in a large bowl. Add oil or butter and whisk well.

2. Mix together all the dry Ingredients: in a bowl and add to the egg mixture little by little, whisking each time.
3. Add more milk if you find the batter too thick. Add a tablespoon at a time and whisk.
4. Place a nonstick skillet over medium heat. Grease the pan.
5. Pour about ¼ cup batter on the pan. Slightly swirl the pan so that the batter spreads.
6. Cook until the underside is golden brown. Flip sides and cook the other side too.
7. Repeat steps 45 with the remaining batter. It makes about 67 pancakes
8. Serve with yogurt and fresh fruits.

Rise And Shine Sweet Bulletproof Coffee Smoothie

Ingredients:

- 3 tbsp. of coconut flakes (optional)
- 1 cup of ice cubes
- 2 organic bananas
- ½ cup of Bulletproof Coffee of choice
- ¼ cup of coconut milk, or almond

Directions:

1. Put all of the Ingredients: into a blender and blend until the mixture is completely even.

Classic Shrimp Ceviche

Ingredients:

- 1 tomato, fresh and thinly sliced
- 1 onion, small in size and finely chopped
- 1 teaspoon of red pepper flakes, crushed
- ¼ cup of lemon juice, freshly squeezed
- 3 tablespoons of butter, grass fed variety and soft
- 1 cup of shrimp, peeled and deveined
- 1 cucumber, small in size, fresh and finely chopped
- 1 avocado, fresh, peeled, pitted and thinly sliced
- 1 jicama, small in size, peeled and finely chopped

Directions:

1. First place your butter into a large sized skillet placed over medium heat.
2. Once your butter is fully melted add in your shrimp and cook for the next 3 minutes or until pink in color and fully cooked through.
3. Then use a large sized salad bowl and add in your cooked shrimp.
4. Fresh cucumber, fresh jicama, fresh avocado, chopped onions and crushed red pepper flakes. Stir until thoroughly combined.
5. Pour your fresh lemon juice over your entire mixture and toss thoroughly to combine. Serve right away and enjoy.

Unomelet Bulletproof Diet Style

Ingredients:

- 1 head OF broccoli, large in size, sliced into florets AND finely chopped
- 1 egg yolk, raw
- 1 tbsp. C8 mct oil
- 1 tbsp. OF lemon juice
- Dash OF sea salt for taste
- Dash OF rosemary, fresh AND for taste

Directions:

1. The first thing that you will have to do is steam your vegetables and once they are fully steamed, drain them well.
2. After that you will need to pour some hot water into your blender to preheat it slightly. Once your vegetables are ready remove the

hot water from the blender and add in your veggies. Next add in the rest of your Ingredients:.

3. Allow your vegetables to cook your eggs as you blend them on the lowest setting until you have an extremely creamy sauce.
4. Pour into a serving dish and sprinkle with your herbs and sea salt for taste. Enjoy.

Celery Cauliflower Smoothie

Ingredients:

- 1 cup coconut milk
- 1 tablespoon raw almonds
- 4 ice cubes
- 2 celery stalks
- 1 cup cauliflower florets

Directions:

1. Mix all the Ingredients: in a blender until smooth and creamy.
2. Pour the drink in glasses and serve it as fresh as possible.

Fat Bombs

Ingredients:

- 5 g grated coconut
- 5 g coconut oil, for chocolate
- 50 g bitter chocolate (dark)
- 50 g unsalted butter
- 150 g cream cheese
- ½ lemon, juice and zest

Directions:

1. Prepare 12 small silicone molds or line a 20x20 cm (8x8 ") square mold with parchment paper, to facilitate demoulding.
2. Melt the butter and coconut oil in the microwave, at intervals of 15 sec. Add the cream cheese and mix well. Add the lemon

juice and zest and the grated coconut, mix. Spread the mixture in the mold.

3. Melt the chocolate and coconut oil in the microwave at 15 second intervals. Spread over the cream cheese mixture.
4. Refrigerate until solid, about 1 hr.
5. Unmold onto a work surface and remove the paper. Cut into squares to obtain 12 pieces.

Moroccan Style Grass Fed Lamb With Sweet & Sour Sprouts

Ingredients:

- 2 cups, Brussel sprouts, halved
- Juice of 1 lemon
- 2 table spoon honey
- Salt and pepper to taste
- 1 ½ pounds grass fed lamb shoulder, boned
- 1 onion, diced
- 2 clove garlic, minced
- Thumb sized piece of ginger, minced
- 2 tablespoons Moroccan 7 spice.

Directions:

1. Add the lamb, onion, ginger, garlic and 7 spice to the slow cooker and cook on low heat for 6 hours.
2. Once the lamb is cooked, pull apart with a fork and set aside.
3. Lightly boil the Brussel sprouts in water with and drain. Toss with the honey, lemon juice and salt and pepper.
4. Serve alongside the lamb. Drizzle the honey and lemon juices around the plate.

Cinnamon Bulletproof Coffee

Ingredients:

- 1 tbsp butter
- 1 tbsp MCT oil
- 2 tbsp weighty cream
- 1 cup newly prepared coffee
- 1 tsp cinnamon powder

Directions:

1. Mix every one of the fixings until smooth and fill a mug. 2. Serve warm.

Baked Burgers

Ingredients:

- 2 lbs. ground beef (if not grassfed, use lean)
- 2 tsp. ground turmeric
- 1 T dried rosemary
- 2 T dried oregano
- Sea salt (to taste)
- 4 slices bacon

Directions:

1. Preheat oven to 325 degrees F. Make about 8 burgers.
2. Combine the spices and rub them directly onto the burgers. Salt to taste.
3. Put a halfslice of bacon on top of each burger and put them on a flat baking pan with sides.
4. Bake for 1520 minutes to desired doneness.

Zucchini Casserole

Ingredients:

- ¾ cup coconut oil or grass fed ghee
- 1 ½ teaspoons dried basil
- 4 pasture eggs, beaten
- Salt to taste
- Pepper powder to taste
- 12 cups zucchini, diced
- 1 red bell pepper chopped
- 1 yellow bell pepper, chopped
- 1 green bell pepper, chopped
- 1 cup quinoa, cook according to the instructions on the package

Directions:

1. Preheat the oven to 350 F.
2. Grease a baking dish with butter generously.
3. Add zucchini, bell peppers, quinoa, coconut oil, basil, eggs, salt and pepper to a bowl.
4. Transfer into the greased baking dish.
5. Spread all over.
6. Bake in a preheated oven at 350 degree F until top is golden brown.
7. Serve hot or warm.

Healthy Banana Bulletproof Coffee Smoothie

Ingredients:

1 ¼ cups of frozen organic bananas, chopped

¾ cups of cold Bulletproof Coffee

¼ cup of raw organic milk

1 tsp. of heavy cream

Directions:

1. Add all of the Ingredients: into a blender and blend until the mixture is smooth.

Easy Ground Beef Salad

Ingredients:

- 1 Cucumber, Fresh and Sliced Thinly
- 2 Avocados, Peeled, Fresh and Pitted
- ¼ Cup of Vinegar, Apple Cider Variety
- ¼ Cup of Lemon Juice, Freshly Squeezed
- ¼ Cup of Oil, Coconut Variety and Fully Melted
- ½ Cup of Cilantro, Fresh and Roughly Chopped
- Dash of Salt, For Taste
- 1 Cup of Beef, Lean and Ground
- 1 tablespoon of Cayenne Pepper
- 3 teaspoons of Lime Juice, Freshly Squeezed

- 2 Tablespoons of Butter, Grass Fed Variety and Soft
- ½ Cup of Red Cabbage, Fresh and Finely Shredded
- 2 Cups of Spring Greens, Fresh

Directions:

1. First brown your beef. To do this use a large sized skillet and set over medium heat.
2. Add in your beef and cook for the next 5 minutes or until thoroughly brown in color.
3. Then add in your butter, dash of cayenne pepper and fresh lime juice.
4. Season with a dash 0f salt and remove from heat. Season with a dash of salt.
5. Next place your avocados, apple cider vinegar, fresh lemon juice, fresh cilantro and coconut oil into a blender.

6. Blend on the highest setting until smooth in consistency. Remove and set aside for later use.
7. Place your vegetables and beef into a large sized salad bowl.
8. Pour your avocado dressing over the top and toss thoroughly until combined. Serve right away and enjoy.

Classic Bulletproof Eggs Benedict

Ingredients:

- 2 eggs, softly poached
- Some hollandaise sauce
- 1 tbsp. Of butter, unsalted and grass fed
- 1 avocado, ripe
- 3 handfuls of spinach, washed and drained
- Dash of sea salt for taste

Directions:

1. Using a medium sized pan, add in your spinach with about 2 Tbsp. of Water.
2. Sauté your spinach until slightly wilted.
3. Then strain the water from your pan and add in your butter and salt.

4. Continue to sauté until the butter is fully melted. Place your spinach onto a serving plate.
5. Place your poached eggs on top of your spinach and drizzle with a touch of hollandaise sauce.
6. Serve with a slice of fresh avocado and enjoy.

Avocado Strawberry Smoothie

Ingredients:

- 1 cup coconut milk
- 1/2 cup coconut water
- 1 teaspoon erythritol
- 1 small avocado, peeled and pitted
- 1 cup fresh strawberries, hulled

Directions:

1. Mix all the Ingredients: in a blender and pulse until smooth.
2. Pour the drink in glasses and serve it as fresh as possible as it tends to lose nutrients in time.

Keto Bread

Ingredients:

- 4 g salt
- 75 ml cider vinegar
- 6 egg whites
- 375 ml boiling water
- 300 g almond powder
- 90 g psyllium husks, very finely ground
- 10 g baking powder

Directions:

1. Preheat the oven to 175 ° C / 350 ° F. Oil a bread pan or a cookie sheet, depending on the cooking Directions: chosen.
2. In a bowl, mix the dry Ingredients:.

3. Add egg whites and apple cider vinegar to the dry Ingredients: and mix for a few seconds using a mixer.
4. Pour the boiling water into the bowl and mix well with the mixer, until the mixture thickens.
5. Transfer the dough to the bread pan and place in the center of the oven.
6. Bake for 7590 min, until bread is golden brown and well cooked inside.
7. Alternatively, divide the dough into 16 balls to form panini.
8. Transfer to the baking sheet, place in the center of the oven and bake for 6075 min.
9. Let the bread cool completely, then slice.

Hand Dived Steamed Scallops With Ginger And Spring Onion

Ingredients:

- Juice of 1 lime
- 2 table spoon coconut oil
- Sea salt to taste
- 68 hand dived scallops
- 1 tablespoon fresh ginger, sliced thinly
- ¼ cup spring onions, sliced thinly

Directions:

1. Place scallops in bamboo steamer with the ginger on top and cook for around 4 minutes.
2. To serve garnish with spring onions and pour the lime juice and coconut oil on top.

Vegan Bulletproof Coffee

Ingredients:

- 1 cup newly prepared coffee
- 2 tbsp coconut oil
- 1 oz natural cocoa margarine (edible)
- 2 tbsp almond butter
- ¼ cup almond milk

Directions:

1. Add every one of the fixings into a blender and cycle until smooth.
2. Serve in a glass.

Creamy Cauliflower

Ingredients:

- ½ tsp. apple cider vinegar
- Your herbs of choice
- Sea salt (to taste)
- ½ head of cauliflower, broken into flowerets
- 3 T grassfed butter
- 2 T coconut oil, melted

Directions:

1. Steam the cauliflower until tender. Put about twothirds into serving bowl and
2. The remaining third into a blender (or bowl if using a hand blender). Add the
3. Remaining Ingredients: and blend until smooth.
4. Pour the blended mixture back

5. Over the cauliflower in the serving bowl.

Shakshouka

Ingredients:

- 4 cloves garlic, minced
- 1 ½ teaspoons paprika
- 1 ½ teaspoons cumin powder
- ¼ teaspoon chili powder
- Pepper to taste
- Salt to taste
- 2 tablespoons cilantro, chopped
- 8 pastured eggs
- 1 ½ tablespoons grass fed ghee
- 4 medium tomatoes, chopped
- 1 large onion, chopped
- 1 small green bell pepper, chopped

- 1 small red bell pepper, chopped
- 2 Serrano peppers, chopped

Directions:

1. Place a large skillet and place it over medium heat. Add ghee to it.
2. When ghee melts, add onions and sauté until light brown.
3. Add garlic and Serrano pepper and sauté for a couple of minutes until fragrant.
4. Add bell peppers and lower heat. Cook until bell peppers are soft.
5. Add spices and sauté for a few seconds until fragrant. Do not let the spices burn.
6. Add tomatoes and simmer until sauce thickens. Add salt and stir.
7. Make 8 small cavities in the sauce at different places in the skillet.
8. Break an egg into each of the cavities.

9. Sprinkle salt and pepper. Cover and simmer until the eggs are cooked.
10. Cook the eggs as per your desire.
11. Garnish with cilantro and serve.

Organic Fruit Bulletproof Coffee Smoothie

Ingredients:

- 24 ice cubes
- 1 ½ cups of yogurt of choice
- 1 tsp. of cinnamon
- 1 cup of fresh brewed Bulletproof Coffee of choice, chilled
- 1 med. organic banana, peeled and chopped
- 1 tbsp. of raw honey

Directions:

1. Brew a fresh cup of Bulletproof Coffee of your choice first.
2. Place the Bulletproof Coffee and the chopped organic bananas in the freezer to chill for at least 10 minutes and no more than 20.

3. After you remove the Bulletproof Coffee and organic bananas from the freezer, add them into a blender along with the remaining Ingredients:.
4. Blend the mixture until it is completely even and smooth.

Simple Egg Salad

Ingredients:

- 1 cucumber, small in size and sliced
- 1 avocado, fresh, peeled, pitted and sliced
- 2 tablespoons of oil, coconut variety
- 1 teaspoon of thyme, fresh
- 2 eggs, hard boiled variety and finely chopped
- Dash of salt and pepper, for taste
- 2 cups of salad greens, mixed
- 1 red bell pepper, seeded and sliced
- 1 yellow bell pepper, seeded and sliced
- ½ cup of tomatoes, cherry variety and cut into halves

Directions:

1. Use a small sized bowl and add in your coconut oil, fresh thyme and dash of salt and pepper. Stir thoroughly to combine.
2. Then use a large sized bowl and add in your mixed salad greens, sliced cucumber, halved tomatoes, chopped peppers and fresh avocado. Toss to thoroughly combine.
3. Pour your oil mixture over your salad and toss to coat.
4. Serve with a topping of your chopped eggs and enjoy right away.

Wholesome Baked Grapefruit With A Touch Of Cinnamon

Ingredients:

- Dash of cinnamon, organic
- sprinkle of nuts, organic and your personal choice
- 1 grapefruit, medium in size and organic

Directions:

1. Slice your grapefruit in half using a serrated knife.
2. Then slowly loosen the sections of the grapefruit as carefully as possible.
3. Next place your grapefruit pieces onto a baking sheet.
4. Make sure that you sprinkle each slice with a generous amount of cinnamon and finely chopped nuts.

5. Set your oven to broil and place your grapefruit slices into the oven.
6. Broil for the next 4 to 6 minutes or until the tops of the grapefruit slightly brown.
7. Remove from oven and serve immediately.

Lemon Cucumber Smoothie

Ingredients:

- 1 cup coconut water
- 1 tablespoon erythritol
- 1 tablespoon MCT oil
- 1 large cucumber
- 1 lemon, juiced
- 1/2 teaspoon lemon zest

Directions:

1. Mix all the Ingredients: in a blender and pulse until smooth.
2. Pour the drink in glasses and serve it as fresh as possible.

Avocado Recipe Stuffed With Cream Cheese And Nuts

Ingredients:

- 5 ml walnut oil
- A few sprigs of chives
- The juice of half a lime
- Salt pepper
- 1 ripe avocado
- 40 g fresh cheese
- 20 walnut kernels

Directions:

1. To make this recipe, start by finely chopping the chives and then crush the nuts.

2. Then open the avocado in half and remove the stone. With a spoon, take a little avocado flesh to leave more room for stuffing.
3. In a salad bowl, mix together the avocado flesh, fresh cheese, crushed nuts, chives, walnut oil and lemon juice. You must obtain a homogeneous filling but not a boiled appearance. Salt and pepper to your liking.
4. Finally, place this stuffing in each of the two avocado halves and enjoy immediately.
5. This recipe is ideal as part of the ketogenic diet since it provides a concentrate of highquality fatty acids. Indeed, avocado is a source of Omega 9 while walnut oil and walnuts are two invaluable sources of Omega3. The stuffed avocado is therefore a concentrate of energy to start the day off right and boost the brain and metabolism.

Spanish Style Mussel And Hake Stew

Ingredients:

- 1 teaspoon saffron
- ½ cup parsley
- Juice of 1 lemon
- 4 tablespoon virgin olive oil
- 5 cups fish broth
- 2 large fillets of Hake, cut into squares
- 1 pound hand dived mussels
- 2 onions, diced
- 3 clove garlic, diced
- 1 tablespoon pimenton

Directions:

1. In a deep frying pan, start by lightly frying the onion and garlic in the olive oil.
2. Add the pimenton and cook for a further 4 minutes.
3. Add the fish broth and saffron and bring to boil.
4. Lower the heat and place the Hake in carefully.
5. Add the lid and cook on a low heat for around 10 minutes.
6. Remove the lid and add the mussels, close the lid and cook for a further 4 minutes.
7. To serve, garnish with the parsley and a squeeze of lemon.

Iced Vegan Bulletproof Coffee

Ingredients:

- 1 cup coconut milk
- 1 tbsp MCT oil
- 2 tsp coconut oil
- 1 cup newly fermented espresso, chilled
- ½ tsp vanilla extract
- 1 tbsp without sugar maple syrup
- Ice blocks for serving

Directions:

1. Pour every one of the fixings aside from the ice 3D shapes into a blender and cycle until smooth.
2. Divide the ice 3D squares between 2 glasses and pour the beverage on top.

3. Serve immediately.

'Whatever' Stove Top Dinner

Ingredients:

- 1 'green zone' meat
- 12 'green zone' vegetables, chopped
- Spinach or kale
- Your choice herbs/spices

Directions:

1. Put some coconut oil in a pan on medium heat. Lightly brown the meat and then
2. Add the veggies and your leafy greens. Sprinkle in your spices and herbs. Stir,
3. Cover, and let it cook until veggies are tender, usually 1015 minutes.

Thai Breakfast Scramble

Ingredients:

- 6 eggs, well beaten
- 1 teaspoon chili powder
- A large pinch freshly ground black pepper
- 2 tablespoon fresh cilantro, chopped
- Salt to taste
- 2 scallions, sliced
- 2 teaspoons fresh ginger, peeled, minced
- 4 teaspoons coconut oil or grass fed ghee
- 4 small garlic cloves, minced

Directions:

1. Place a skillet over medium high heat. Add coconut oil.

2. When oil is melted, add ginger, garlic, and scallions.
3. Stirfry for a few seconds until fragrant and add beaten eggs.
4. Scramble the eggs by stirring constantly and cook until the texture you desire is achieved.
5. Sprinkle salt, chili powder, and pepper powder.
6. Add cilantro. Mix well.
7. Remove from heat and serve.

Sweet Banana Bulletproof Smoothie

Ingredients:

- ¼ cups of raw honey
- 1 organic banana, chopped
- 1 cup of ice cubes
- 1 cup of raw organic milk
- 2 tbsp. Bulletproof coffee

Directions:

1. Add all of the Ingredients: into a blender and blend until the mixture is even and smooth.

Skinny Peppermint Mocha Smoothie

Ingredients:

- 1 teaspoon of Stevia
- 2 Stevia Peppermint Drops
- Heavy cream
- Chocolate flakes, up to 1 dash
- 1½ cups of Bulletproof Coffee of choice, frozen
- ½ cup of raw organic milk,
- 2 teaspoons of unsweetened cocoa powder

Directions:

1. Gather all of the Ingredients: and add them into a blender.
2. Blend the mixture until it is smooth.

Simple Scrambled Eggs With Zucchini

Ingredients:

- 1 egg, large in size and beaten
- Dash of salt and pepper, for taste
- 2 teaspoons of lard, grass fed variety
- 1 zucchini, fresh and thinly sliced

Directions:

1. The first thing that you will want to do is place your lard into a medium sized skillet placed over medium heat.
2. Once your lard has fully melted add in your zucchini to your skillet and cook for the next 5 to 10 minutes or until it is tender to the touch.
3. Once tender spread onto an even layer in your skillet.
4. Then pour your beaten egg over your zucchini.

5. Cook while stirring occasionally until firm to the touch.
6. Season with a dash of salt and pepper before removing from heat.
7. Serve right away and enjoy.

Filling Early Morning Beef Patties

Ingredients:

- 1 tbsp. Of thyme, fresh and organic
- 1 tbsp. Of rosemary, fresh and organic
- 1 tbsp. Of coconut oil, organic and extra virgin
- 2 pounds of beef, ground and grass fed
- 1 tsp. Of sea salt for taste

Directions:

1. Preheat your oven to 350 degrees.
2. Then using a large size mixing bowl, combine your beef, freshly ground herbs and dash of sea salt.
3. Using your hands mix your Ingredients: thoroughly until mixed well.
4. Then form your mixture into thick sized patties.

5. Next, grease a medium sized baking pan with some coconut oil and cook your patties for the next 25 to 30 minutes or until they are thoroughly cooked through.

Cauliflower Watercress Smoothie

Ingredients:

- 1 tablespoon lemon juice
- 1 cup coconut water
- 1 tablespoon MCT oil
- 1 1/2 cups cauliflower florets
- 1 cup watercress
- 1/2 avocado

Directions:

1. Combine all the Ingredients: in a blender and pulse until smooth.
2. Pour the smoothie in serving glasses and serve it as fresh as possible.

Raspberry Chia Seed Pudding

Ingredients:

- Frozen raspberries 60g
- Erythritol / Stevia 10g
- Unsweetened coconut milk 120g
- Chia seeds 40g

Directions:

1. Mix the coconut milk and chia seeds. Flavor with cinnamon, a few drops of vanilla extract or orange blossom
2. Book in the fridge for 2 hours
3. Meanwhile thaw the raspberries
4. Add the raspberries over the pudding, sprinkle with stevia / erythritoltype sweetener if needed and enjoy

Beef Carpaccio, Hazelnuts & Egg Yolk Dressing

Ingredients:

- 1 teaspoon honey
- ½ cup rocket leaves
- Salt and pepper to taste
- 6 tablespoon virgin olive oil
- 2 pounds of grass fed beef fillet
- ¼ cup hazelnuts, crushed
- 2 pastored egg yolks
- Tablespoon apple cider vinegar

Directions:

1. Slice the fillet of beef into thin slices and bat out between two sheets of cling film.
2. Lay the beef so it covers the whole plate.

3. In a bowl add the egg yolk and slowly whisk in the oil to emulsify.
4. Add the honey vinegar and salt and pepper.
5. To serve sprinkle the hazel nuts and rocket leaves over the beef and drizzle the dressing around the plate.

Salted Caramel Bulletproof

Ingredients:

- 1 tbsp grasstook care of salted butter
- 1 tbsp weighty cream
- A touch of salt
- 1 cup newly prepared coffee
- 1 tbsp lowcarb caramel sauce
- 1 tbsp coconut oil

Directions:

1. Process every one of the fixings in a blender until velvety.
2. Serve the beverage in a mug and enjoy.

Pumpkin Spice Bulletproof Coffee

Ingredients:

- 1 cup newly prepared coffee
- 2 tbsp weighty cream
- 1 tbsp butter
- 1 tbsp MCT oil
- 1 tbsp pumpkin puree
- 1 tsp pumpkin zest powder
- ½ tsp cinnamon powder + something else for topping
- ½ tsp vanilla extract
- 2 tsp erythritol
- Whipped cream for topping

Directions:

1. Add every one of the fixings aside from the whipped cream to a blender and interaction until smooth.
2. Pour the beverage into a cup, twirl a few whipped cream on top and embellishment with some cinnamon powder.

Creamy Broccoli Soup

Ingredients:

- 4 c bone broth or veggie broth
- ½ c grassfed butter
- Sea salt to taste
- 68 cups broccoli florets
- 34 shallots, minced
- 1 carrot, sliced

Directions:

1. Put a dab of butter into a large stockpot and lightly sauté the shallots and carrot.
2. Add the broccoli and cook until it's bright green.
3. Pour in the broth and continue to cook until broccoli is tender.

4. Add the remaining butter and blend (a hand blender works well) until desired consistency. Season with sea salt and serve hot.

Brussels Sprout Hash

Ingredients:

- 4 eggs
- 3 teaspoons coconut oil
- 2 tablespoons grass fed butter
- Salt to taste
- Pepper powder to taste
- 10 large Brussels sprouts, halved
- 1 onion, sliced
- 1 large sweet potato, chopped
- 6 grape tomatoes

Directions:

1. Place an ovenproof skillet over medium heat.

2. Add coconut oil and butter. When the butter and oil melts, add sweet potatoes and onion and sauté for a while until slightly tender.
3. Add Brussels sprouts, salt and pepper and sauté for another 5 minutes.
4. Add tomatoes and sauté for a couple of minutes.
5. Remove from heat and crack eggs over it. Sprinkle salt and pepper.
6. Place the skillet in a preheated oven and bake at 350 degree F until eggs are set to the consistency you desire.

Honey Mocha Smoothie

Ingredients:

- 1 tablespoon of cocoa powder, unsweetened
- 1½ teaspoon of raw honey
- 2 to 4 ice cubes
- ¾ cup of brewed Bulletproof Coffee
- 1 ¼ cup of raw organic milk of choice

Directions:

1. Add all of the Ingredients: together in a small sauce pan.
2. Mix them together until they are warm then add them into a blender with 1 cup of ice.
3. Blend the mixture until it is even and smooth.

Spicy Bacon Wraps

Ingredients:

- ¼ teaspoons of black pepper, for taste
- ¼ teaspoons of garlic, powdered variety
- 2 teaspoons of hot sauce, your favorite kind
- 12 slices of bacon, thick cut
- 2 avocados, fresh, peeled, pitted and cut into slivers
- ¼ teaspoons of chili, powdered variety

Directions:

1. Wrap each of your avocado slivers with your bacon and place onto a lightly oiled baking sheet.
2. Season these wraps with your powdered garlic and dash of black pepper.

3. Place your baking sheet into your oven to bake for the next 20 minutes at 425 degrees.
4. After this time remove from your oven and transfer your wraps to a large sized serving platter.
5. Sprinkle your favorite hot sauce over the top and powdered chili. Serve while warm and enjoy.

Early Morning Breakfast Salad

Ingredients:

- Dash of Sea Salt For Taste
- A Small Dab of Coconut Oil, Extra Virgin
- 1 Avocado, Ripe and Organic
- 1 Broccoli Floret, Fresh and Organic
- 1 Carrot Stick, Fresh and Organic
- 1 Celery Stick, Fresh and Organic
- 2 Eggs, Large In Size and Pastured
- 5 Ounces of Baby Spinach, Fresh and Organic

Directions:

1. Using a vegetable peeler to remove the carrot peelings on the carrot.
2. Then, cut your carrot into tiny pieces and place the pieces into a large sized salad bowl.

3. Next, cut up your celery and place it in the salad bowl.
4. Then, remove the central part of the avocado, slice it up into small sized pieces.
5. Next place the avocado into the salad bowl as well.
6. Next dice up your baby spinach and broccoli.
7. Place your broccoli into a pot of boiling water and boil your broccoli for about 5 to 7 minutes.
8. Then add in your spinach and boil it until it wilts.
9. This should take about 2 to 3 minutes. Remove from pot and set aside to cool.
10. Once fully cooled, place both your boiled spinach and broccoli into your salad bowl along with your other vegetables.
11. Then prepare your eggs in any way that you like using your coconut oil.

12. Top your salad with your eggs and season with your dash of sea salt.
13. Toss gently and serve immediately. Enjoy.

Savory Egg Muffins

Ingredients:

- ¼ cup of green onions, fresh, organic and finely chopped
- Dab of coconut oil, organic and extra virgin
- 12 eggs, large in size and pastured
- Dash of sea
- ¼ cup of cilantro, organic, fresh and finely chopped

Directions:

1. Preheat your oven to 350 degrees. While it heats up lightly grease a muffin tin with a generous amount of oil or butter.
2. Next chop up your cilantro and onions. Set aside.

3. Whisk your eggs using a large sized mixing bowl and add in your sea salt.
4. Then stir in your cilantro and onion mixture.
5. Mix your muffin batter until thoroughly combined and pour into your muffin tins.
6. Place into your oven to bake for the next 20 to 25 minutes or until the eggs are fully set.

Coconut Carrot Smoothie

Ingredients:

- 1/2 cup fresh coconut flesh
- 1/4 cup cashew nuts, soaked overnight
- 1 pinch cinnamon powder
- 1 carrot, sliced
- 1 cup coconut milk

Directions:

1. Combine all the Ingredients: in a blender and pulse until smooth.
2. Pour the drink in glasses and serve it as fresh as possible.

Tropical Cilantro Smoothie

Ingredients:

- 1 cup fresh tangerine juice
- 1/4 cup raw almonds
- 1 tablespoon MCT oil
- 1 cup fresh cilantro
- 2 slices fresh pineapple
- 1 cup coconut water

Directions:

1. Mix all the Ingredients: in a blender and pulse a few minutes until smooth and creamy.
2. Pour the drink in glasses and serve it as fresh as possible.

Bulletproof Coffee

Ingredients:

- Coconut oil 10g
- UnSalted butter 20g
- Black coffee 200g

Directions:

1. Run a large black coffee
2. In a shaker, mix the coffee with the butter (or the whole cream) and the coconut oil
3. Sweeten if necessary with a sweetener like Stevia or erythritol

Keto Raspberry Smoothie

Ingredients:

- 250 ml cold tea
- 100g raspberries
- 125 ml coconut milk

Directions:

1. In a blender, mix all the Ingredients:!
2. Served fresh

Trout And Avocado Lettuce Wraps

Ingredients:

- 4 tablespoon grass fed full fat yoghurt
- Salt and pepper to taste
- 1 head of baby gem lettuce
- 2 fillets of trout
- 1 large avocado, peeled and cubed
- Juice of 1 lemon
- 2 scallions, finely chopped
- ¼ cup flat leaf parsley

Directions:

1. Place the trout fillets in the bamboo steamer and cook for around 5 minutes.

2. In a bowl combine the avocado, scallions, parsley, yoghurt, lemon juice and salt & pepper. Flake the cooked trout into the bowl.
3. Mix well so the yoghurt coats all the Ingredients:.
4. Peel back the baby gem lettuce so you get small petal like cups.
5. Fill each cup with the filling and enjoy!

Red Onion Squash Soup

Ingredients:

- 6 cups vegetable broth
- 1 cup organic grass fed cream
- ½ cup grass fed butter
- Salt and pepper to taste
- 1 pound red onion squash, peeled and cubed
- 2 onions, diced
- 2 clove garlic, sliced
- 1 sprig of fresh thyme

Directions:

1. In a large sauce pan bring the butter to a medium heat.
2. Add the onion, garlic and thyme and cook gently for 10 minutes.

3. Add the squash and vegetable broth. Bring to the boil.
4. Cook for around 30 minutes.
5. Transfer to a liquidizer and blend until smooth.
6. Once smooth, add the cream, salt and pepper.
7. Serve hot!

S’mores Flavored Bulletproof

Ingredients:

- 1 tbsp butter
- 1 tbsp sans sugar S’mores syrup
- 1 cup newly fermented coffee
- 1 tbsp MCT oil

Directions:

1. Process every one of the fixings in a blender until smooth.
2. Fill serving glasses and enjoy.

Iced Bulletproof Coffee With Peanuts

Ingredients:

- 2 tbsp sans sugar maple syrup
- Whipped cream for topping
- 2 tbsp squashed toasted peanuts
- 1 cup newly fermented coffee
- 1 tbsp MCT oil
- 1 tbsp butter
- 2 tbsp unsweetened cocoa powder

Directions:

1. Except the whipped cream and peanuts, add every one of the fixings to a blender and interaction until smooth.

2. Pour the beverage into a glass, whirl a few whipped cream on top and embellishment with the peanuts.
3. Enjoy!

Greek Lemon Shrimp

Ingredients:

- 3 eggs
- 2 lemons
- 1 T MCT or olive oil
- 2 c shrimp
- 1 c chopped leeks
- ½ c chopped celery
- ½ c chopped carrot

Directions:

1. In a large fry pan, cook the leeks, celery, and carrot over low heat for 510 minutes.
2. Add the shrimp (fresh or thawed) and a little water to form a broth. In a bowl, beat the eggs until frothy.

3. Continue beating the eggs as you add in the juice from the lemons and then the oil.
4. Turn off the heat under your fry pan. Remove a little hot broth from the pan and beat it into the lemon/egg mixture.
5. Pour the mixture into the fry pan and stir. Garnish with parsley and serve.

Sausageburger Balls

Ingredients:

- 1 egg
- Oregano or basil (to taste)
- ½ Lb. Spicy sausage or chorizo
- ½ lb. Ground beef

Directions:

1. Preheat oven to 325 degrees F. In a large bowl, mix all the ingredients.
2. Form the mixture into bitesized minimeatballs.
3. Cook in a flat baking dish with sides until desired doneness is reached, about 1015 minutes.

Smoked Salmon Frittata

Ingredients:

For Smoked Salmon Frittata:

- 1 tablespoon grass fed ghee or coconut oil
- 78 ounces smoked salmon
- 8 large pasture eggs

To Serve:

- 1 green onion
- Green onion sauce as required

Directions:

1. Preheat the broiler.
2. Slice the green onion.
3. Add eggs to a bowl and beat the eggs with an electric mixer until light and fluffy. Set it aside.
4. Take an ovenproof skillet and place it over medium heat. Add ghee.

5. When ghee melts, add eggs and cook until the middle part is runny and sides are slightly set.
6. Place the smoked salmon on the eggs. Remove from heat.
7. Place the skillet under the broiler and cook until the eggs are set.
8. Remove from the oven. Garnish with green onions and serve with green onion sauce.

Bulletproof Bread

Ingredients:

- 12 pasture eggs
- 2/3 cup MCT oil or coconut oil, melted
- ½ teaspoon sea salt
- 1 ½ cups coconut flour
- 1 teaspoon ground flax
- 2/3 cup apple sauce

Directions:

1. Add coconut flour, ground flax, applesauce, eggs, coconut oil to a bowl and stir. Using a hand blender, blend until smooth batter is formed.
2. Grease 2 small loaf pans and line with parchment paper.

3. Pour batter into the pans. Place the pans in an oven.
4. Bake in a preheated oven at 350 degree F for about 45 minutes.
5. Remove from oven and cool completely. Run a knife all around the edges of the bread and invert on to a plate.
6. Slice each loaf into 22 slices.
7. Fill with toppings of your choice and serve.

Protein Pumpkin Spice Bulletproof Coffee Smoothie

Ingredients:

- 2 tablespoons of cinnamon
- 1 tablespoon of ground ginger
- ½ tablespoon of allspice
- ½ tablespoon of ground cloves and nutmeg
- ½ tablespoon of ground nutmeg
- 12 ounces of Bulletproof Coffee, freshly brewed
- 1 scoop of vanilla protein powder, or of choice
- 1 tablespoon of pumpkin puree
- ½ teaspoon of homemade pumpkin pie spice mix

- 2 to 4 ice cubes

Directions:

1. Add all of the Ingredients: into a blender and blend until the mixture is smooth.

Gingerbread Spiced Bulletproof Bulletproof Coffee Smoothie

Ingredients:

- 1 tbsp. of coconut oil, organic can be used
- 1 tsp. of Stevia, or raw honey (Optional)
- 2 to 4 ice cubes
- 1 tsp. of organic gingerbread spice mix (
- 1 tbsp. of grassfed butter, or almond butter

Directions:

1. Combine the gingerbread spice mix with the Bulletproof Coffee grounds then brew the mixture.
2. Add the hot Bulletproof Coffee into a blender along with the remaining Ingredients:.
3. Use caution and blend the mixture until it is smooth.

Delicious Smoked Salmon And Avocado

Ingredients:

- 1, 1 pound of salmon, smoked variety and wild sockeye variety
- Dash of sea salt, for taste
- 1 avocado, fresh and peeled

Directions:

1. First slice up your avocado into thin strips along with your salmon.
2. Then wrap your avocado slices onto a piece of salmon. Repeat until all of your salmon has been wrapped.
3. Season with a dash of your sea salt and serve right away.

Bulletproof Friendly Cupcakes

Ingredients:

- Dash of Salt, Himalayan Variety
- 6 Eggs, Large in Size and Separated
- 2 teaspoons of Vanilla, Powdered Variety and Mold Free
- 1 teaspoon of Cocoa Powder
- 1 tablespoon of Flour, Sweet Rice Variety
- 6 Tablespoons of Erythritol
- 6 Tablespoons of Xylitol
- 12 Ounces of Chocolate, Dark Variety
- 1 ½ Sticks of Butter, Unsalted Variety and Grass Fed Variety

Directions:

1. The first thing that you will want to do is preheat your oven to 350 degrees. While your oven is heating up line two muffin pans with muffin liners.
2. Add your Erythritol and xylitol into a blender and pulse until finely ground. Set this mixture aside for later use.
3. Then use a small sized saucepan and add 2 cups of water into it. Simmer over low to medium heat.
4. Next add in your chocolate and butter into a large sized bowl. Place this bowl directly over your water and allow to heat up until completely heated through. This should take at least 10 minutes. Remove from heat and allow to cool slightly before serving.
5. Use a stand mixer and add in your Erythritol mixture, dash of salt and egg yolk. Blend on

the medium to high setting until your mixture is thick in consistency.

6. This should take at least 3 minutes.
7. Fold your egg mixture into your melted chocolate mixture.
8. Add in your vanilla, cocoa powder and flour. Fold again to incorporate.
9. Use a separate bowl and add in your egg whites. Beat with an electric mixer until soft peaks begin to form.
10. Add into your Erythritol mixture and continue to beat until peaks begin to form. Add in your chocolate mixture and fold again until combined.
11. Spoon at least ¼ cup of your batter into your muffin cups.
12. Place into your oven to bake for the next 25 minutes.

13. Remove and allow to cool for the next 5 minutes before transferring to a cooling rack. Enjoy whenever you are ready.

Fruity Health Bars

Ingredients:

- ½ cup of honey, raw
- ¼ cup of coconut oil, extra virgin and organic
- 1 tsp. Of cinnamon, ground and organic
- 2 cups of shredded coconut, unsweetened and organic
- ½ Tsp. Of sea salt, for taste
- 3 cups of assorted nuts, of your choice and organic
- 1 cup of cranberries, dried and organic

Directions:

1. Place some parchment paper into a medium sized baking dish and set aside.

2. Then pour your assorted nuts into a large sized mixing bowl and combine thoroughly.
3. Next take one cup of your assorted nut mixture out of your bowl and place them onto a medium sized cutting board. Chop up your nuts into fine pieces.
4. Then take your remaining two cups of assorted nuts and place them into a blender or food processor. Pulse the nuts until they are chopped to a small enough size that they can be put into your fruit bars.
5. Then, add all of your nuts from both your food processor and cutting board back into your mixing bowl. Toss with your hands to thoroughly combine.
6. Next add in your dried cranberries and shredded coconut to your mixing bowl. Stir thoroughly to combine your mixture until mixed well.

7. Using a small sized saucepan add your coconut oil, cinnamon, sea salt, and honey. Cook your mixture over medium to low heat, making sure that you stir until your mixture begins to bubble slightly. Once your mixture begins to bubble remove it from heat.
8. Next pour your liquid over your nut mixture in your mixing bowl. Stir thoroughly to combine until everything is evenly mixed.
9. Once mixed well pour all of your Ingredients: into your baking dish.
10. Then use a second sheet of parchment paper and firmly press it over your mixture until it is well packed together. Let your mixture sit for about two hours. Then, cover and place into your freezer to freeze for at least one or two hours.
11. Then use your parchment paper to take the granola mixture out of your baking dish as gently as possible. Transfer your granola onto

a small sized cutting board. Next using a sharp knife, slice your granola into thin bars. Set aside and save your granola for whenever you are ready to enjoy them.

Filling Scrambled Eggs With A Side Of Asparagus

Ingredients:

- ¼ cup of spinach, baby, fresh and packed lightly
- 1 onion, medium in size, white and diced finely
- Dash of sea salt and pepper for taste
- 4 strips of bacon fat, pastured
- 1 ½ cups of bell pepper, any color, fresh, peeled, deseeded and finely diced
- 4 eggs, large in size and pastured
- 1 tomato, medium in size and diced finely

Directions:

1. Preheat your oven to 350 degrees.

2. While your oven heats up use a medium sized skillet or sauce pan, start cooking your bacon strips over medium heat. Be careful that you don't crisp them. Make sure that you leave them a little raw.
3. Next add in your diced onions, tomatoes and peppers and sauté them in the pan with the bacon for at least 7 minutes or until they start to cook through. Set aside.
4. Then take out a medium sized bowl and crack your eggs into it. Beat them lightly and season them with your salt and pepper.
5. Then take a cup cake baking tray and line the cups with silicone baking cups. Spoon your bacon and vegetable mixture in each cup, making sure to fill each cup halfway.
6. Next take your bowl with the eggs and pour the beaten eggs on top until the cups are almost full.

7. Place them into your oven to bake for at least 17 minutes in the oven or until the eggs are set. Remove from oven.
8. Take out one cupcake sized omelet and serve immediately. Enjoy.

Cilantro Limeade Smoothie

Ingredients:

- 1/2 teaspoon grated ginger
- 1 1/2 cups coconut water
- 1/4 cup cashew nuts, soaked overnight
- 1 cup fresh cilantro
- 1 lemon, juiced

Directions:

1. Mix all the Ingredients: in a powerful blender.
2. Pulse until smooth and creamy.
3. Pour the drink in glasses and serve it as fresh as possible.

Ginger Pineapple Smoothie

Ingredients:

- 1 cucumber, sliced
- 1 cup coconut water
- 1 tablespoon MCT oil
- 4 slices fresh pineapple
- 1 teaspoon grated ginger

Directions:

1. Combine all the Ingredients: in a powerful blender or food processor and pulse until smooth and creamy. It might take a few minutes.
2. Pour the drink in glasses and serve it as fresh as possible.

Keto Pancake

Ingredients:

- Egg 106g (4 medium eggs)
- Odourless Coconut Oil 10g
- Unsalted butter 10g
- Almond powder 30g
- Whipped Cheese 30g

Directions:

1. Heat the coconut oil in the microwave
2. In a bowl beat the eggs and add the whipped cheese and almond powder
3. Heat a pan with a knob of sweet butter
4. Eat salted with a fried egg or sweetened with a Franky's type sugarfree syrup

Zucchini Soup

Ingredients:

- Zucchini 100g (1/2 zucchini)
- Thick fresh cream 30% 60g
- Dijon mustard 10g

Directions:

1. Blanch the sliced zucchini in boiling water for 10 minutes
2. Mix with the crème fraiche and the mustard
3. Season and serve

Asparagus Soup

Ingredients:

- 1 cup organic grass fed cream
- Juice of 1 lemon
- 3 cups baby spinach
- 5 tablespoon virgin olive oil
- Salt and pepper to taste
- 5 cups asparagus
- 2 onions, chopped
- 2 clove garlic, chopped
- 5 cups vegetable broth

Directions:

1. In a large saucepan bring the olive oil to a medium heat.

2. Add the onion, garlic and cook gently for around 10 minutes.
3. Add the vegetable broth and bring to a boil.
4. Add the asparagus and cook for 4 minutes.
5. Stir in the spinach and immediately transfer to a liquidizer.
6. Blend until smooth then add the cream, lemon juice, salt and pepper.
7. Serve Hot!

Vietnamese Beef Soup

Ingredients:

- 1 pound grass fed beef brisket
- 2 cups Pak Choy
- 1 stick cinnamon
- Thumb sized piece of ginger
- 1 cup scallions
- ½ cup cilantro leaves
- 5 cups beef or chicken broth
- 2 hot green chilies
- 2 tablespoon fish sauce
- Salt and pepper to taste

Directions:

1. Apart from the Pak Choy and cilantro, combine all the Ingredients: into a large sauce pan and bring to the boil.
2. Cook for around 2 hours or until beef can be pulled apart by a fork.
3. Add the Pak Choy and cook for a further 5 minutes.
4. To serve add the cilantro leaves.

Iced Peppermint Bulletproof Coffee

Ingredients:

- 1 tbsp MCT oil
- 2 drops peppermint extract
- Ice blocks for serving
- 1 cup newly prepared coffee
- 2 tbsp weighty cream
- ½ tsp erythritol

Directions:

1. Blend every one of the fixings aside from the ice solid shapes in a blender until smooth.
2. Spoon some ice 3D squares into a serving glass and pour the beverage on top.
3. Enjoy!

Bulletproof Coffee Popsicles

Ingredients:

- 1 cup almond milk
- 1 (13.5 oz) can coconut
- 1/3 cup erythritol
- 1 tbsp coffee powder
- ¼ tsp nutmeg powder
- 3 tbsp MCT oil

Directions:

1. Process every one of the fixings in a blender until creamy.
2. Pour the combination into 8 popsicles hills and freeze for somewhere around 4 hours.
3. Appreciate when ready.

Coconutcrusted Chicken

Ingredients:

- Fresh parsley
- Dried oregano
- 1 lb. chicken, cut into strips
- 2 eggs
- Shredded unsweetened coconut flakes or powder
- Sea salt

Directions:

1. Preheat oven to 325 degrees f.
2. Mix the coconut, salt, parsley, and oregano in one bowl.
3. In another bowl, beat the eggs until well blended.

4. Dip the chicken into the egg and then roll in in the dry mix until coated. Bake until it starts to brown.

Salmoncuke Bites

Ingredients:

- Cucumber, cut into ½ inch pieces
- Sea salt
- Smoked salmon

Directions:

1. Cut the salmon into strips, and wrap each strip around a piece of cucumber (or
2. zucchini or avocado). Season with salt or salad dressing (as desired).

Winter Vegetable Salad

Ingredients:

- 1 small head cabbage, cored, cut long strips of 1 inch width
- 1 teaspoon each of fresh rosemary, thyme and oregano chopped
- ¼ cup almonds, chopped
- 4 teaspoons apple cider vinegar
- Salt to taste
- 4 slices thick cut pastured bacon
- 12 teaspoons high quality olive oil
- 8 teaspoons bulletproof Brain Octane oil or MCT or coconut oil

- 1 pound each of parsnip, carrots, turnip, winter squash and sweet potatoes, chopped into 1 inch pieces

Directions:

1. Place bacon on a baking sheet that is lined with parchment paper.
2. Bake in a preheated oven at 320 F for 10 minutes. Do not brown it. Only cook it.
3. Remove the bacon. When cool enough to handle, crumble and set aside.
4. Let the bacon fat remain on the baking sheet.
5. Add the vegetables to the baking sheet and pour Brain Octane oil, 8 teaspoons olive oil, salt, and fresh herbs. Toss well.
6. Bake for about 20 minutes.
7. Add cabbage and toss. Bake until vegetables are tender.
8. Remove from the oven and transfer into a large serving bowl.

9. Pour the remaining oil over it. Sprinkle vinegar, bacon, and almonds and serve warm.

Avocado And Salmon

Ingredients:

- Sea salt to taste
- 8 ounces cold smoked wild sockeye salmon or 2 cold smoked wild sockeye salmon of about 4 ounces each
- 2 Hass avocadoes

Directions:

1. Peel the avocadoes. Remove the seed and discard it. Slice each of the avocadoes into 4 slices of ¼ inch thickness.
2. Place the salmon on your work area. Slice the salmon into 8 slices or each of the 4 ounces salmon into 4 slices each.
3. Place an avocado slice on one salmon slice. Sprinkle salt over it. Wrap the salmon over the avocado. Serve.

Bulletproof Coffee Creamsicle Smoothie

Ingredients:

- 1 cup of ice, or less
- 2 ounces of organic orange juice, freshly squeezed
- 3 ounces of brewed Bulletproof Coffee, chilled
- 8 ounces of vanilla almond milk, or of choice

Directions:

1. Combine all of the listed Ingredients: into a blender and blend until the mixture is smooth.

Nutritional Bulletproof Coffee Smoothie

Ingredients:

- 1 tablespoon of cocoa powder, unsweetened
- 1 sm. chopped organic banana, frozen
- 1 teaspoon of chia seeds
- 8 ounces raw organic milk
- 1 ounce of brewed Bulletproof Coffee, chilled

Directions:

1. Combine all of the Ingredients: into a blender and blend until the mixture is even and smooth.

Smoked Salmon And Eggs

Ingredients:

- 4 tablespoons of ghee, grass fed variety and fully melted
- 1 teaspoon of dill, fresh
- Dash of salt, for taste
- 4 eggs, pastured variety and poached
- ½ cup of salmon, smoked variety and wild caught variety

Directions:

1. First heat up your ghee in a large sized skillet placed over medium heat. Once your ghee is fully melted add in your dill and cook for at least 30 seconds. Remove from heat.
2. Place your smoked salmon among two serving plates.

3. Top off with your poached eggs and cooked dill.
4. Season with a dash of salt and serve right away. Enjoy.

CPSIA information can be obtained
at www.ICGtesting.com
Printed in the USA
LVHW080001061222
734629LV00016B/1205

9 781990 120848